Living With Your Pain

A Self-Help Guide To Managing Pain

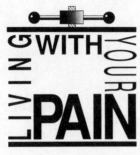

Annabel Broome
Dudley Health Authority

& Helen Jellicoe
Wandsworth Health Authority

The British Psychological Society
in association with Methuen

First published in 1987 by The British Psychological Society, St Andrews House, 48 Princess Road East, Leicester, LE1 7DR in association with Methuen & Co. Ltd, 11 New Fetter Lane, London EC4P 4EE.

British Library Cataloguing in Publication Data.

Broome, Annabel
  Living with your pain: a self-help guide to managing pain
  1. Anesthesia   2. Analgesia
  I. Title II. Jellicoe, Helen
    III. The British Psychological Society
  616'. 0472 RD82

ISBN 0-901715-77-8

Set in Bembo by Arrow Photoset, Leicester.

Printed and bound in Great Britain by A. Wheaton & Co. Ltd, Exeter.

CONTENTS

Introducing ourselves

All the people described in this book have learnt to enjoy life in spite of pain. Whether your pain is from an old injury, arthritis, 'wear and tear', an infection like shingles, or a bad scar, the approach described here will help you understand and cope with your pain.

No doubt, you will already have found your own ways of coping, so we start from the basis that you are the expert on your pain. This book builds on your expertise.

It is based on the questions pain sufferers ask and describes the solutions they find useful. These personal solutions, plus the wealth of research into self-help methods, form the basis of our programme.

Who are we?

Both of us are clinical psychologists working with pain sufferers. Annabel Broome has researched, written and lectured internationally on pain and now works with pain sufferers and those who treat them. Helen Jellicoe works closely with a variety of health service professionals to encourage better understanding and care of people with chronic pain. We have seen people in their own homes, in out-patient clinics, in specialist pain clinics and in hospital. Their problems have all been different, and between them they have had every conceivable sort of treatment. But one fact stands out above all others: the most effective changes come about when people begin to solve their problems for themselves.

Who is this book for?

The book is a practical guide for you to follow week by week. It is designed for people who are still in pain despite full medical investigation and a range of treatments. Unfortunately, not all pain can be cured and some people are left with frequent or even permanent pain. Pain killers can reduce pain, but for many they do not help, and for some the idea of taking pills for ever is not acceptable.

You may be one of the many people who cannot be cured and have been left to cope on their own. But you may still be in doubt and think your doctor can do more for you. If so, go and see your doctor before starting our programme, because this is for people who have accepted that there is no cure, and know that they have to learn to live with their pain.

Coming to terms with your pain

We wish that there was always an easy way to take your pain away, but very often there just isn't.

Our own work with pain sufferers tells us that the first important decision is recognizing that you are stuck with the problem and have to make the best of it. The second stage is to get to understand the pain better so that you can take control. This book assumes that you have made the first decision, and are now ready for the programme to take you through a step-by-step system to manage your pain.

This is the programme which you will follow:

▶ **Week One:** You will note how your pain varies through-out the day.

▶ **Week Two:** You will begin problem-solving; you will be testing out reasons for variations in your pain.

▶ **Week Three:** You will see how much relaxation can help, both when you are practising specific exercises, and also when you are out and about.

▶ **Week Four:** You will be examining the relationship between your everyday activities and your pain. You will begin to try out changes and make adjustments. This prob-lem-solving will be the foundation of your plans for the future.

The programme does not give all the answers, but it will help you ask the right questions, so that you can build up your own unique way of tackling your difficulties.

You and the medical services

One of the problems most often expressed to us by pain sufferers is their difficulty in dealing with medical services. Because so many people need help with this, Chapter 6 suggests how to get the best information and the best service from the medical profession. This is important, as you need accurate medical information to start planning realistic changes.

The practical programme in this book is firmly based on research findings. Chapter 7 outlines current thinking on the psychology of pain, and relates this research to the programme in Chapters 2–5.

At the end of the book is a list of addresses of societies, organizations and groups which can offer help, information and contacts.

1. How do you feel about your pain?

▶ Who do you believe?
▶ The importance of other people
▶ Putting on a brave face
▶ Why carry on?
▶ You're the expert
▶ Helping yourself

We have developed our programme by working closely with pain sufferers on their problems.

One of the biggest obstacles is feeling helpless and frustrated and unable to do anything about it, but the fact that you are reading this book suggests that already you think some improvements are possible. This is a positive first step. So many of the pain sufferers we see feel passive and helpless, and it is difficult for them to make the switch to take active measures to find a better way of living. As psychologists working with pain sufferers, we are more and more convinced that it is the will to cope that really matters.

Although you may not have this problem of helplessness, people looking for help to cope better with their pain and distress have a lot in common.

To get this point across, let's describe some of the people we know and the things they most often say when we meet for the first time. You can judge for yourself how similar their experience is to your own.

66 Has something been missed? 99

Sandra has frequent back and leg pain. She tried to describe it to her friends, her family and her doctor, but was never sure that they really

Clearly, someone who believes their backache may be cancer is going to feel many times more anxious than someone who believes it is due to a fall on the ice.

So, Sandra's fears were making her anxious and depressed, and this increased her suffering.

When Sandra came to see us we spent some time helping her prepare a list of the questions she wanted answered by her medical advisors. It was only when she had a clear idea of what was wrong that she could start to calmly take stock, and make realistic plans for the future.

Once she was reassured and had a clearer understanding of her pain, she was able to start this planning.

❝All the family have really had to pull together but we'll try anything to get her back put right.❞

When Elsie hurt her back the doctors told her to rest. So, she'd been taking it easy, but she still found it hurt even after two years. Her family were 'golden': they did everything for her in the house to let her rest, and they had taken her to visit specialists all round the country, to try to get her back put right.

Elsie was hoping that one day someone would have the magical cure, and everything would then get back to normal.

When Elsie came to see us, she was annoyed at our suggestion that she could learn to cope better. What she really wanted was a cure. In spite of her doctor saying this was now very unlikely, she still believed that if only the right technique could be found, the pain could be taken away.

But there is always uncertainty surrounding pain problems. Pain sufferers often hope there might be a medical cure, if only it could be found.

Elsie was cure-seeking, despite the evidence that no more could be done medically. Meanwhile, she and her family had adopted a way of living that looked after her as an invalid. All the family needed to change if Elsie was to have any chance of getting back to a normal life. As things stood, the rest of the family were, unfortunately, ensuring that Elsie remained dependent. She could only start taking control of her life again if the family gave her the opportunity and space to build up her own independence.

When Elsie wanted to start cooking again, it took her nearly three hours just to prepare the vegetables – it would have been much quicker for one of the others to do it, but much better for Elsie to start doing it herself and build up her strength again.

So Elsie had to make it clear to her family how much she wanted to try. She convinced them that it was better for her to gradually build up her stamina and her interests as she took the first steps back to normality and coping with pain.

The reactions of important people around us can be extremely influential. The only way others know you are in pain is by your behaviour. There is no thermometer to show how much pain you are in; it's a private experience, but people will assume from the way you sit, walk, take pills or lie down that you are hurting.

You know yourself that some people are more concerned when you obviously have pain than when you appear to be coping well and are putting a brave face on it.

Maria, a young housewife married to a very busy executive, found that when she was in a lot of pain, her husband took a lot more care of her, and spent more time with her.

It is easy to see how tempting it might be for her to show a little more pain behaviour to remind others that all is not well.

Every pain sufferer has to look very carefully at the messages they are giving out, and ask whether the important people around them are really helping them regain control.

3

❝I try as best I can to put a brave face on it, and carry on as normal for as long as I can.❞

On good days Sandra would wake up and think of all the things that needed doing in the house. She would rush around tidying up, washing, ironing, cleaning windows and so on. By the end of the day she was feeling stiff and aching all over. But in spite of that she would soldier on and prepare the family's evening meal, making sure they were settled before she took herself to bed with a hot water bottle and a couple of pain killers. The next day she was good for nothing.

Sandra, like many, had an all-or-nothing approach: doing as much as she could when she felt good, until she hurt so much she was unable to do anything at all. The effects of this activity sometimes cost her two or three days in bed. She was trying to fight the pain and often carried on regardless of extreme discomfort. She worried that family and friends would think her a nuisance, a moaner, or a hypochondriac if she took things easy. She felt obliged to battle on, trying to show she was still capable of being a good wife and mother.

Once Sandra had decided things weren't going right she examined the situation carefully. She realized that she had got to learn to pace her life, so she could get all the jobs done that were important to her, but she spread them out carefully across the day. This kept her pain at manageable levels, and although Sandra still has some way to go, she feels she is beginning to get to grips with the pain without letting her family down.

❝What's the point?❞

It can be so painful to do things that it seems a natural reaction to do less and less. But this can lead to other problems. Getting out of touch with work, friends, hobbies and interests gradually takes away all the fun in life. As it becomes increasingly difficult to meet friends and they stop calling, sufferers feel more isolated and trapped by the pain. They have lost most of the good things in life and become increasingly helpless, irritable and depressed.

Bob was a 41-year-old electronic engineer, married, with two children. He realized that nothing more could be done to cure his back pain, caused by a car accident four years before. "I have to take so much time off work, I'm worried if they're going to keep me on. I'm irritable with the family and I can't make any plans. I can't do any of the things I used to enjoy."

Bob felt trapped and miserable with his pain and as he withdrew more, so he became more depressed. As he got lower, so he felt like doing things even less. He was in a vicious circle. When we first met Bob, he had nearly given up. He felt a failure.

When he saw other fathers out playing with their children he was reminded of the days when he was fit and strong, when he could just jump into the car and go out for the day, play football with his friends, or simply sit watching TV with his family. He dwelt on the differences between then and now, and felt he'd lost everything worthwhile. He was disappointed and resentful, with nothing to look forward to.

Bob had a difficult time when he first came to see us. He felt powerless to make changes, angry at what had happened, and angry that we did not seem to understand how awful his life was. Gradually, he realized that the will to change had to come from him. He realized how much he had withdrawn into himself, and that life was passing him by. He began to use his training as an engineer to examine his problem in more detail and test out some solutions. He redesigned his driving seat, joined the PTA at his son's school and helped the older children in their model-making club.

Bob is feeling less controlled by the pain: he knows now that he can make changes, and is treating it as a challenge. Increasing his activity was difficult and did hurt at first, because he had become so inactive, but each small achievement gave him a huge boost of confidence.

Active participation is the linchpin of any programme. No one can do this for you.

66 You can't teach me anything about pain. I've been coping with it for years. 99

This may be true for you, and many of the people who come to us quite rightly resent the suggestion that they could cope better. They are quick to point out that they *are* copers, and they have had to live with their pain for some years, which takes some doing.

People find their own ways of coping, and some work well.

John, who suffered severe arthritic pain, coped with this quite differently in two situations. At his daughter's wedding he distracted himself by getting absorbed in the events and people around him. In the privacy of his own home, however, he sits quietly alone in a comfortable position reminiscing on pleasant events in his past.

It is important to have a range of strategies, because different things will work at different times. It's not a simple matter of finding one method that works; it's necessary to have a range of methods to choose from, which will work for you on different occasions, and with different levels of pain.

You must be ready to help yourself

You will see, as you work through the programme, that your own expertise and your willingness to try out different solutions is the key to getting the best out of life. We cannot tell you what to do, but we can help you understand your problems more clearly and test out ways of dealing with them.

Although the programme runs in a particular sequence, you may find you need to backtrack occasionally to earlier sections such as the relaxation exercises. For instance, it may be that as you start to increase activity you need to re-learn the more specific techniques for relaxing.

Don't be afraid to use the programme at your own pace and in your own way.

Good Luck!

2. Getting to know your pain

▶ How to record your pain
▶ What recording tells you
▶ Preparing for the next stage

It is a common belief that paying attention to pain makes it worse and you will often have been told 'If you didn't spend so much time thinking about it and got out and did something you'd not feel the pain so much'.

Many of our patients have tried to get on and keep busy in spite of their pain. But in spite of carrying on regardless they are having a fairly miserable and painful time.

Although this attitude is admirable, it is more useful to gradually build up a profile of your pain, gathering detailed information. This will help you understand how to do more without hurting more. Week One of the programme shows you how to record your pain and find out how and why it varies at different times.

Taking note of your pain

Your first task is to spend a week recording the amount of pain you feel over the day. This does not mean dwelling on your pain for hours – it means estimating how much it hurts at different times.

Start by recording the pain you have now.

You can record both how bad the pain is and how bad it is at different times of the day.

1. Make a cross at that point on the vertical line which you think best describes the pain you are feeling at the

moment. (A cross towards the bottom means no pain, a cross towards the top means the pain is at its worst.) With practice you will get better at judging how far along the line your pain is at any given moment.

Try it now.

The worst it ever is

No pain

2. You can also record changes in the amount of pain you have during the day by giving it a number from 0-5 at the times given on the chart. (A score of 0 means no pain, and a score of 5 means the worst it ever is.)

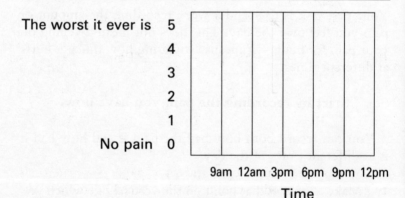

The worst it ever is   5
4
3
2
1
No pain   0

9am 12am 3pm 6pm 9pm 12pm

Time

8

This is all you need to do for the first week. Simply record the amount of pain you feel at different times during the day. You can choose to record your pain in any way you like, either every hour, every four hours, at meal times or any other regular time to suit you. However, recording pain levels more than once every two hours is likely to be unnecessary and inconvenient.

What recording can tell you

Most people we meet at the pain clinic insist that there is no variation to their pain; it just hurts all the time. But when they record it in this sort of detail over the day they are surprised to find that they feel different amounts of pain at different times.

For many people pain increases throughout the day with a high point at about 8.00 pm. People who are at home most of the time tend to feel higher levels of pain, and these people usually have pain more of the time. But these are average figures. Remember that each person will have their own pain pattern. You will need to find out your own.

These graphs show three quite different patterns of pain across the day.

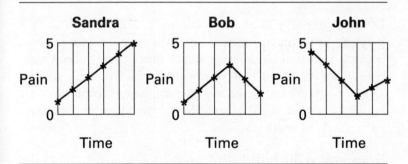

Sandra's pain builds up during the day. This pattern is typical of somebody who gradually becomes more tense during the day and battles on in spite of the pain.

Bob's pain, on the other hand, starts quite low and builds up to a peak at the middle of the day. It reduces as the day progresses but never gets as low as it was in the morning. His pain is at its highest after he has spent three or four hours sitting at a drawing desk at work. He cannot really recover from this as he has the stress of driving home and being with his young family in the evening.

John's pain is very high in the early morning, plummets during the day, and then rises slightly during the evening. This is fairly typical of someone with arthritic pain. Their joints are stiff and painful on waking but gradually ease with use during the day.

What have I learnt in week one?

Is there a daily pattern?

Compare your daily pattern with Sandra's, Bob's and John's and see if you can offer any explanation for your good and bad times. (Your daily patterns may not be very obvious from one day's recording, so wait until you have recorded your pain over seven days before you try to identify a clear pattern.)

Is there a weekly pattern?

Don't worry if you are not able to identify a typical daily pattern. Your recording will not have been a waste of time, because you will have learnt many other things about your pain. You may find that your pain varies from day to day, and you may have a weekly pattern where some days are regularly worse than others. Some people find Saturdays worse, others work days.

Does my pain build up?

You may find that your pain builds up steadily to a peak then stays bad for a while, even for a few days. Alternatively, your pain may come on suddenly and wear off gradually.

10

Have I got more than one pain?

You may have learnt to distinguish more than one type of pain. For instance, you may find that you have one pain which you describe as a dull ache and another, quite different, stabbing pain. If so, then you will need to record each type of pain separately. If you have two pains then you can use a different symbol on a single chart for each one. Mark your chart with a cross for one pain and a dot for the other, or use different coloured pens.

Vera suffered two types of facial pain. Her daily recordings are shown below. The knife records the level of her cutting pain and the mallet records the level of her dull ache.

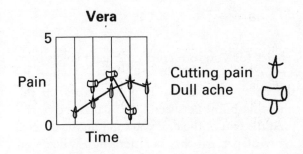

Does activity make it worse?

While you are recording you may begin to notice which activities tend to make it worse. Note these down for later on.

Where do I go from here?

Looking at your pain in this way is useful because you are learning more and therefore you can make more educated attempts to help yourself. The knowledge you have gained from this first week will help towards a full analysis of your pain and help you plan ahead.

Already you may have begun to appreciate how and why your pain varies. One of the main effects will be from daily activities.

> *Sandra found, after only one week's recording, that certain things like cleaning the windows made her back bad for hours. She limited herself to doing only a few minutes of a job, and then resting. In this way she did much more, but in smaller bursts of activity. Most importantly of all, her pain never reached the peaks it used to.*

In addition to activity, your thoughts and mood, along with any tension and stress you are feeling will all be having some effect on your pain. Having learned how to record and describe your pain accurately, the next step is to make a much more thorough assessment of why it varies.

Pain diary

Here are seven charts for you to record your pain levels over a week. By doing this you will get a picture showing the changes over the course of the week. Put a cross on the upright 'time' line on a point between 0 (no pain) and 5 (the worst it ever is). At the end of the day you can join the crosses up and see the sort of pattern that is emerging. When you have completed the seven charts you will have a record of changes during the week. A sample chart has been completed for you so that you can see what to do. Use a pencil to do your recording, then you can repeat the exercise after following the programme.

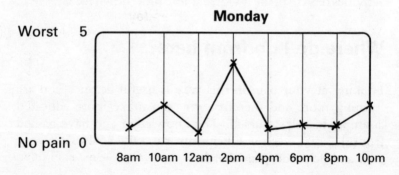

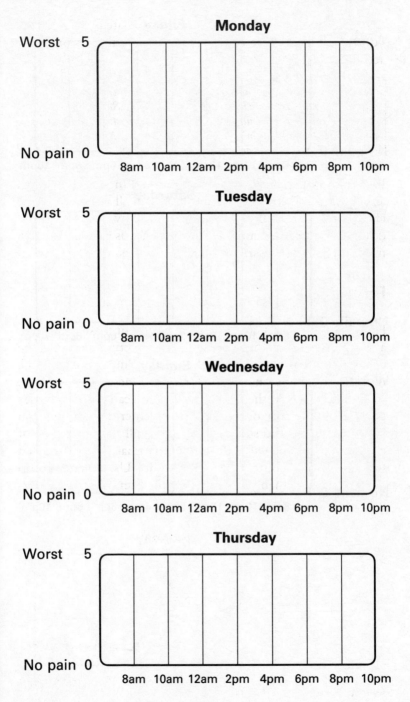

Monday

Worst 5

No pain 0

8am 10am 12am 2pm 4pm 6pm 8pm 10pm

Tuesday

Worst 5

No pain 0

8am 10am 12am 2pm 4pm 6pm 8pm 10pm

Wednesday

Worst 5

No pain 0

8am 10am 12am 2pm 4pm 6pm 8pm 10pm

Thursday

Worst 5

No pain 0

8am 10am 12am 2pm 4pm 6pm 8pm 10pm

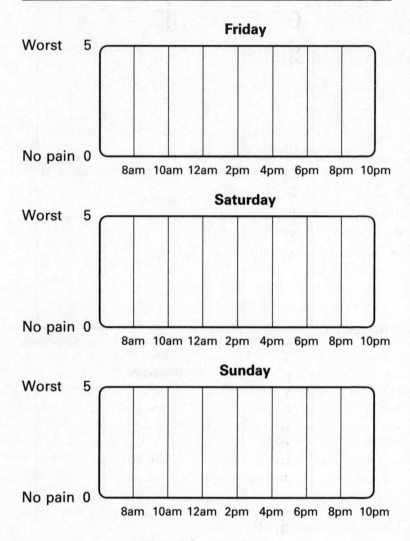

3. Tension and pain – the vicious circle

▶ What causes tension?
▶ Getting out of bad habits
▶ Psychological tension
▶ Creating your own tension
▶ Recording your tension
▶ What you will learn in Week Two

One of the most familiar words of advice when you are in pain is *'RELAX'*. This often causes offence because what it suggests is not simply that the pain is caused by tension, but that you are largely responsible for how tense you are and therefore you are causing the pain yourself. This is only a breath away from saying that it is 'all in the mind'.

There is no question that pain gets worse as tension increases but the relationship between pain and tension is not so simple, because the pain itself causes tension.

The vicious circle

You can recognize times when you become worked up by the pain, feeling frustrated because it will never go away. This feeling of being trapped is a sure sign that you are caught in a vicious circle where pain and tension are fuelling each other.

Whatever the cause of the tension it can result in a vicious circle – the tension makes the pain worse, which then makes you more tense and so on.

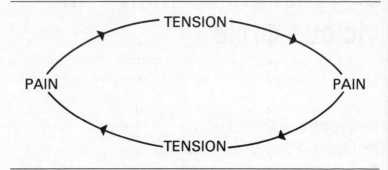

What is causing tension?

To prevent being overwhelmed in this way it is important to be clear about what is making you tense and to take preventive action before it leads you into the downward spiral.

Tension can affect us both physically are psychologically. We will deal with these two sources of tension separately, but remember that in reality they occur together. This means that, in practice, if you are feeling 'uptight' or stressed you will also find that your body is tense.

Physical tension

Physical signs of tension show themselves most commonly in the muscles, which become tense and tight. You may also notice faster breathing and quicker heart rate. In extreme tension (panic) physical signs include sweating, wobbly legs, light-headedness, 'butterflies' in the stomach, and palpitations. People with a long and painful medical history can get these panicky feelings just at the thought of visiting a doctor, or the dread of a hospital visit.

Muscle guarding

Physical tension, especially muscle tension, is common because when we are in pain we tend to hold our bodies very rigid and in unusual postures to try to protect the painful areas. Limping, sitting sideways, or holding the spine in a

16

lopsided way are some of the ways in which pain sufferers try to 'get comfortable'.

This is called 'muscle guarding'. Unfortunately, far from alleviating pain, it usually makes matters worse because it causes tension and discomfort elsewhere in the body.

> *Brian suffered severe phantom limb pain after losing a toe in an accident; he held his leg unnaturally stiff and walked on the outside of his foot to avoid walking on the painful area. As a result he not only had foot pain, but also suffered severe pain in his knee.*

The uneven body postures caused by muscle tension and guarding strain different muscles and joints which, in turn, begin to hurt. Guarding can also leave muscles unused. These become wasted as time goes on and it hurts when trying to use them again.

Start monitoring your physical tension by noting any 'guarding' postures you have developed. Make a list of any tensing you do with your body to try to get comfortable or reduce the pain.

Guarding postures

When lying: _____

When sitting: _____

When standing: _____

When walking: _____

Can you think of any others? _____

_____

17

Getting out of bad habits

Now that you recognize how much your pain is affecting your natural posture and movement, try to get out of these habits. It sounds obvious, but if you are sitting in a crouched or unnatural position try to sit up straight. If you are standing lopsided, try to stand straight; if you are limping, try walking evenly.

It may seem impossible at first but have a go. Remember, you may have been guarding your pain in this way for many years, so it will take time to change it. Retrain yourself in easy stages by setting aside some time each day to hold your body in the correct posture and gradually build up the amount of time you spend doing this each day. You may feel odd or self-conscious at first, but people are often surprised at how easy it is to retrain a habitual limp or sit up straight. What you are now doing is getting rid of a long-held habit.

Taking note of physical tension

The next stage is to begin learning how to recognize how tense your body is at different times of the day and in different situations. Take note of your muscle tension at this moment. Are there some tell-tale signs of tension?

- ► Is your jaw clenched?
- ► Are your shoulders slightly raised?
- ► Is your breathing irregular?

Give yourself an overall tension rating from 0 to 5 (where 0 means your muscles feel relaxed, warm and soft; and 5 means they are tight, hard and sore). Write down your estimate:

Muscle tension rating now = ...

Psychological tension

We do not get tense simply because the pain hurts, but also because the pain means something to us. It means different things to different people.

> *Peter's tension, for example, was largely a result of his thoughts about the pain. He only had back pain when he stretched his shoulders backwards. It did not incapacitate him, but he had been to many doctors who were unable to identify what was wrong.*
>
> *The background to his problem was particularly important. Two years previously he had seen many doctors because of chest pain. At first it was believed that he was being 'neurotic', but six months later gall-stones were diagnosed and he had the appropriate operation to remove them. At the time he was advised that if he got a pain in the future he should not let it go undiagnosed. In the light of this experience Peter was more aware than others of pain because for him it signalled something very important and potentially dangerous.*

As a rule, something like a headache does not concern us too much. We may put it down to 'the time of the month', drinking too much, or being tired. But if someone we know has recently been diagnosed with a brain tumour following headaches, then a headache takes on a more sinister meaning. This causes tension and as a result more pain, and more attention will be focused on the pain. You may notice yourself occasionally tensing the local muscles or touching the area to see if the pain is still there.

If you find yourself doing this ask what your pain means to you. To start with try to clarify what it is you think is physically wrong with your body. You may find that your understanding is rather vague: for example, some people with back pain suspect that if they move too much their spine will give way. Consequently, they hold themselves stiff and make only limited movements.

If you do have a rather unclear idea of what is wrong there are two things you can do.

1. You can ask your doctor to explain your physical condition in a way that makes sense to you. (Chapter 6 gives some guidelines for making the most of visits to the doctor.)

19

2. You can also actually test out how much you are able to do, rather than simply assume that you cannot or should not do certain things. (Chapter 4 explains how you can find out your physical limitations without damaging yourself.)

Self-imposed tension

But to many people chronic pain means more than having something physically wrong. They understand precisely what is wrong and are only too aware of the physical limitations that they will have to get used to. For example, arthritis is not something which is simply going to go away, and this can lead to feelings of frustration and despair. Each pain is a reminder of having become disabled. The pain means missing out on many activities that used to be enjoyed. It can mean loss of work, loss of social life, loss of sexual intimacy and loss of self-esteem. Each twinge of pain is a reminder that things will never go back to how they used to be.

If you are getting this distressed, and have even come to dislike yourself and life itself in this way, you are going to kick against these limitations. Your poor self-image creates tension. You are angry that you are in pain and angry with yourself for not being able to do things. As a result you push and force yourself to do things as if nothing is wrong, striving to be a 'normal' person. The tension at this point comes from *self-imposed* pressure.

> Olive put enormous pressure on herself to perform perfectly and 'act as if nothing was wrong'. She was now middle-aged and had suffered back pain since the pregnancy with her second child. She lived in a farmhouse in an isolated area and whenever her daughter and son-in-law came to visit with the grandchildren, she felt much worse than usual. She often felt so much pain that, far from giving them the welcome she would have liked, she had to go to bed.
>
> When Olive began to record her levels of tension over the day it was clear that her tension was building up well before the visit. She was putting pressure on herself to perform well. This made her tense, and the tension was increased still further by the anticipation that she might not feel well, and might have to go to bed as she had done in the past.

Thus, we return to the vicious circle. Frightening thoughts and lowered mood breed tension. This increases the pain, which produces more negative thoughts, depression and more tension. This process is very rapid; it can happen in milliseconds and the result is that you feel totally controlled by the pain.

Taking note of your tension

Before learning to control and reduce tension you need to be able to recognize how tense you are, how this affects your pain, and what is causing your tension. This takes practice, but careful recording saves you jumping to conclusions and assuming that you know what is causing your tension.

Pain and tension record

Date	Tension	Pain	What am I doing?	What am I thinking?
23/3	3	2	Waiting for nurse.	Will she find anything wrong?
24/3	0	1	Just finished some gardening	That was really relaxing.

This is a record form which shows how to record tension. There is a blank form for you to fill in at the end of this section. Note that there are four columns which you have to fill in every few hours. In the first column record how tense you feel. This may be muscle tension, or other physical signs, or it may be just a feeling of being 'wound up'. Rate your tension on a scale of 0 to five (where 0 = *calm and relaxed* and 5 = *as tense as you have ever been*).

In the second column rate how much pain you feel on a scale from 0 to 5. The third and fourth column will give you some idea of what is making you tense. In the third column say what you are doing and in the fourth column say what you are thinking about at the time.

This recording exercise puts together most of the information you need. It should help you to understand:

1.   How pain and tension are related.

2.   How tension is related to what you are doing.

3.   How pain and tension are related to what you are thinking.

Pain and tension record

Date	Tension (0–5)	Pain (0–5)	What am I doing?	What am I thinking?
9am				
1pm				
5pm				
8pm				
11pm				

What have I learnt in week 2?

Do not try to come to any conclusions whilst you are doing the recording, but wait until you have gathered information over a week. When you have this information look at it carefully and see if you can make any links.

Pain and tension

You can plot a graph showing both tension and pain ratings over the day. This graph shows clearly how David's pain and tension levels went together. He found he often had high tension just before an increase in pain. Also, the graph shows that for him the best part of the day for doing things was between 10am and 2pm, when tension and pain levels were lower.

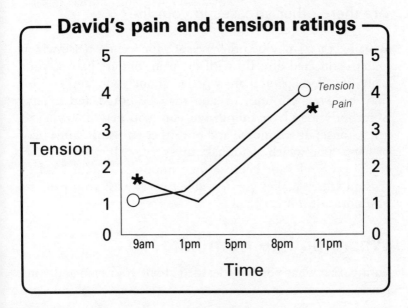

Are there physical causes of tension?

It will be clear to you by now that tension is caused by a variety of things and for each of us the causes vary from day to day. For instance, it may be the result of what we are doing with our bodies – staying too long in one position, taking no exercise, or adopting guarding postures.

Can the way I am thinking cause tension?

At other times your thoughts might be creating tension. Negative and frightening thoughts in particular will cause problems:

'I am never going to cope with this'
'I know something seriously wrong has been missed'
'I know I'll only have to come home again because the pain will be too much to bear'
'There's no point in going. I won't enjoy it. I'll spoil it for everyone. They won't want to be bothered with me again!'

Are there other stresses in your life?

Equally, there may be other reasons for feeling tense which aren't connected directly with the pain, but are part of your daily life. Perhaps you are worried about your family. You may be over-working, or you may be bored and lonely. Somebody may have humiliated you; you may be trying to sell a house; or a hundred and one other stressful things may be happening which go to make up everyday life. These other stresses are relevant because they impose a certain level of tension which makes you less able to deal with your pain; so you notice it more.

Where do I go from here?

Summarize what you have learned about your pain and your tension.

▶ Make a list of all the insights you have gained into yourself from the recordings.

▶ By doing this you are well on the way to gaining some control.

24

You can begin changing things because all the things you have been looking at are under your control. With this information you are in a much stronger position because you are able to put your finger on things that could be changed in your behaviour, your attitudes and your lifestyle.

With a clearer idea of what makes you tense you can begin controlling your tension. For example, you may find that your negative expectations about going out are the major reason you don't go. If this is so then you are in effect telling yourself not to go out. Change might involve exploring why you think this. It could also be a question of telling yourself that you are unlikely to get out at all unless you can begin to look forward to doing so.

How can I reduce tension?

The message of this chapter is *Know Thyself* and at this point we hope that you have started to understand a bit more about your pain. The next two chapters assume that you are now becoming more and more of an expert on yourself. They give practical advice on how to go about making changes which will help you begin to enjoy life in spite of the pain.

Chapter 4 describes ways of reducing physical tension. You can try some of these now if you think that muscle tension is a major problem for you. But remember that relaxation will be of no use to you unless you are able to recognize your tension in the first place.

BE VIGILANT: if you wake feeling 'low' with the pain, just stop and check whether your teeth are clenched. When you stand waiting in a queue, or your appointment is running late, or you sit wondering 'Why did this have to happen to me?', check how tensely you are holding your body. Notice how your body tension waxes and wanes with everyday activities and check how your mood and thoughts are often accompanied by corresponding changes in muscle tension.

Chapter 5 describes how to assess your physical limitations systematically and carefully. It then shows you how to build up activity gradually so that you can resume and maintain a lifestyle which is as full and interesting as you would like.

4. Making changes: Relaxation

▶ How to relax
▶ Muscle relaxation
▶ Breathing exercises
▶ Relaxing as part of everyday life

Knowing how to relax will help you calm down even when you feel a lot of pain or when you get worked up over something. You probably have your own ways of relaxing, perhaps reading a good book, day dreaming, having a hot bath, watching TV, knitting or fishing. These methods are good and should be used if they work for you. But this chapter is more concerned with the deliberate attempts you need to make to train your mind and body to feel as fully relaxed as possible whatever is going on around you.

Relaxation is a skill and it will take a little time and practice to get the hang of it. People who have been using relaxation for many years continue to explore new and more effective techniques.

Why does pain make me tense?

Pain tends to make you tighten up. As explained in Chapter 3 this 'muscle guarding' causes poor posture, which leads to aches and pains in other parts of the body. For instance, someone suffering from neck pain may hold their neck stiffly and carefully to guard from hurting, thus causing stiff neck, stiff shoulders and even tension headaches.

When you have learned how to relax properly you will become more aware of your tension and you can relax at the

27

earliest signs. You will be better able to notice whether you are tensing up unnecessarily in an effort to reduce your pain. You will gradually learn to pace your activites sensibly so that you can do more and at the same time remain calm and in control. Reducing tension through relaxation is one way for you to learn to reduce pain and make the most of life.

If you have worked systematically through the book you will by now have a more detailed picture of your own pattern of pain and tension, and how it changes at different times.

The exercises here should, when you have practised them thoroughly, help you feel calm and in control. The techniques we offer will not suit everybody, and may need some adaptation to suit you better. Nevertheless, they have been developed out of years of work with people in pain who find that once they have learnt relaxation, it becomes a part of everyday life. They find it particularly useful to be able to relax when the pressure is on: when your boss is criticising, when your youngest child is home late, while you are waiting at the dentist or queuing in the post office.

But you need to practise to make relaxation work like this for you.

Relaxation methods

These methods will teach you to reduce tension in the main muscle groups and reduce your general level of arousal. For instance, your blood pressure will go down and your heart will beat more slowly when you are fully relaxed. This is a way of reversing the tension in your body, and just as you have learnt to feel tense so now you will learn to feel relaxed.

How do I start?

1. *It is not easy to begin to learn a new skill.*
    Start learning under the best possible conditions. For example, when the house is quiet, in a room or place where you naturally feel at ease, and make sure you are unlikely to be disturbed. If necessary, put up a *Do not disturb* notice on the door.

2. *Practise the skill.*
   Rather like learning to drive or ride a bike, it will take some time and deliberate practice. Build your practice sessions into your daily routine, so you always remember to do it – for example after lunch, returning from work, or before going to sleep at night.

3. *Choose a key word.*
   This is a word you will use to set up your feeling of relaxation and say as you start the deep breathing, such as CALM, RELAXED, QUIET or EASY.

4. *Start noticing the earlier signs of tension.*
   You will have recorded these in your previous self-monitoring. Start using the measured breathing and your key word, so you can bring on the feeling of relaxation.

5. *Try visualizing with your eyes shut.*
   Some people cannot imagine a scene very clearly at all, but can build up a feeling of being in a calm place by using their other senses like hearing, smell and touch, in their imagination. These are useful skills to help deepen the relaxed feeling and create a pleasurable day dream.

Muscle relaxation

1. Sit or lie as comfortably as you can, loosen any tight clothes, and let your hands fall by your sides with your legs slightly apart. Lie easily and loosely.

2. Take a point to focus your eyes on, until you feel very relaxed. Don't strain your eyes, but concentrate on the spot as you start slow breathing. This will help you concentrate, but as you relax more, you may wish to shut them. That's OK.

3. Breathe in slowly, right down to the bottom of your lungs, holding the breath in for about 6 seconds. Breathe out slowly using your key word. Get a feeling of relief as your breath leaves you.

4. Keeping your breathing slow and regular, start tensing and relaxing your muscle groups. For each muscle group

29

inhale and tense the muscles for about 6 seconds and then breathe out and relax, focusing on the relaxed muscles for a few minutes. Always breathe slowly, deeply, in a relaxed manner, and using your key word on the out-breath. Work through your body in the sequence given in the relaxation exercise on pages 32–35.

5. Now focus for a few minutes on the deep, warm and calm feeling you have created.

6. Enjoy the feeling, and lie there for a while.

How do my thoughts affect my pain?

The way you think about things can also affect your body. If you think angry thoughts, your body tenses up; depressing thoughts will make you feel tired.

If you think calm thoughts you will find this usually relaxes you, but if you think of the last row you had with someone then you will find yourself getting a bit hot and bothered. Thoughts *can* make us tense!

Some people find when they are relaxing that they are still turning things over and over in their minds. Don't get worried about it, it's OK – but try to concentrate mainly on the present, and try to think simply about yourself and your body, as you are the most important focus of this exercise. Turn your attention inwards – things may be going on around you, but they are not important, let them go. Just feel peaceful, and concentrate on the quietness of your breathing.

How visualization can help

Once you can feel relaxed, try to use some visualization. You could imagine a peaceful scene. Choose one you particularly like or remember, possibly by the sea, in the woods, in your garden, or by a log fire. If you are not good at building up a scene visually, then build one up using your other senses – the noises, the smells and the sounds from a scene that makes you feel quite calm.

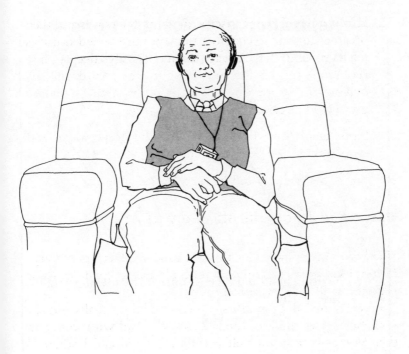

Visualization exercise

▶ Tell yourself you feel heavy, calm and relaxed.

▶ Let your breathing become more shallow, and more easy and automatic.

▶ Keep saying to yourself on the out-breath that you are feeling calm and relaxed by using your own personal key word.

▶ As you begin to imagine a scene in more and more life-like detail so you will begin to take yourself out of your body and into the realms of day-dream and fantasy.

⸺ Relaxation exercise: part one ⸺

Muscle group   Tension procedure

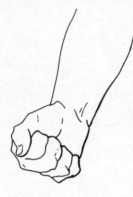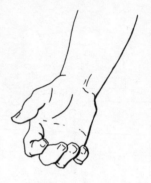

(i) Writing hand and lower arm.   Tense muscles by making a tight fist.

Hold . . . then relax.

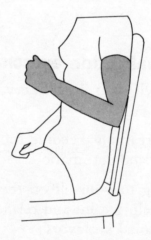

(ii) Upper arm.   Press elbow into back of chair, pushing downwards.

Hold . . . then relax.

(iii) and (iv) Repeat (i) and (ii) for other hand and arm.

Relaxation exercise: part two

(v) Forehead.

Wrinkle up forehead and brow, lift eyebrows.

Hold . . . then relax.

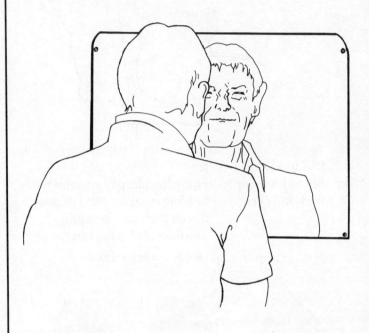

(vi) Nose and upper cheeks.

Clench jaws tightly, wrinkling nose.

Hold . . . then relax.

(vii) Jaws and lower cheeks.

Clench jaws, bite teeth, pull corners of mouth back.

Hold . . . then relax.

(viii) Neck.

Press firmly against back of chair.

Hold . . . then relax.

⸻ Relaxation exercise: part three ⸻

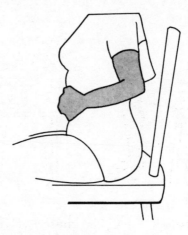

(ix) Shoulders, upper back and chest.   Take slow deep breath and while holding it, sit forward slightly, throw chest out, bringing shoulder blades together.

Hold . . . then relax.

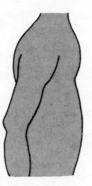 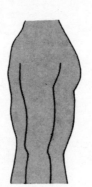 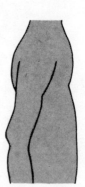

(x) Stomach.   Pull muscles in.
Hold . . . then relax.

Relaxation exercise: part four

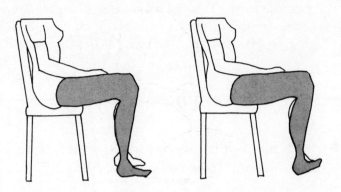

(xi) Right thigh.   Flex muscles if lying down;
                            press heel to floor if sitting.
                            Hold . . . then relax.

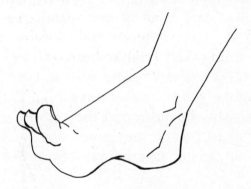

(xii) Right calf.   Pull toes upwards if sitting;
                            point toes away if lying.
                            Hold . . . then relax.

(xiii) Right foot.   Curl toes downwards.
                            Hold . . . then relax.

(xiv) Repeat (xi)-(xiii) for left leg and thigh.

Breathing

Some of you will have noticed rapid and shallow breathing as you become tense. This can cause particular problems by making you feel light-headed and less in control. It needs remedying, so if you have noticed this try a breathing exercise.

Breathing exercise

▶ Sit with your hands clasped together, resting lightly on your stomach.

▶ Start breathing out slowly, letting your stomach fall as you push the air out. Let your lungs fill with air again, your stomach rising as they do so. Use counting to slow down each out-breath. Start with 5 and steadily count down to 0, letting the air out slowly, your stomach falling. Use your key word (for example 'CALM') as you breathe out and just let yourself go as the warm air leaves you. Fill up your lungs slowly and repeat the exercise, each time trying to breathe out more slowly. With practice you can increase the count from 10 to 0.

▶ This deep breathing will help you increase your control, and the counting will stop your breathing becoming more and more shallow and running away with you.

Quick relaxation

After you have taught yourself exercises that suit you and you feel calm and relaxed, you may want to try this quicker version which, when well practised, will help you quickly counteract your tense feelings.

Quick relaxation exercise

► Sit down comfortably in an armchair.

► Shake your legs and arms out and rest them lightly down.

► Check each part of your body to see if it is relaxed (if it is not, work on each tense part, doing tense/relax exercises just as before).

► Start breathing deeply, counting on the out-breath 3 – 2 – 1.

► Use your key word on each out-breath.

► Use your visualized scene to create a sensation of heaviness or warmth drifting upwards from your toes to your head.

► Stay like this for a while, noting the difference.

It may help to get a friend to record a tape of the exercise or even for you to make one yourself, so you don't strain to remember each detail as you are practising.

You must practise!

Even once you have learnt all these skills properly it is essential to keep them well practised. Many people, once they are confident they can do it, stop practising. If you do get out of practice you can simply take yourself back through muscle relaxation (the longer exercise) and build up the skill again. You should be able to learn it again more quickly, since it is a technique you will have tucked away, and will not have lost completely. Just like driving or riding a bike it is better if you keep practising, but it is a skill you can relearn very quickly. It is not quite like starting back at 'square one' again.

Relaxation in everyday life

The aim is to have a practical technique ready for use when you are out and about, so you can continue with what you are doing. To do this you will need to practise until the skill is at your fingertips. You are aiming to be able to feel calm and relaxed in 1 or 2 seconds. By the end of training you should be able to do this by using your key word, by breathing slowly and deeply, and quickly bringing on the whole response you have now taught yourself. This should be useful for any tense moments – going to the dentist, waiting for a bus, or feeling rushed.

John had noticed that when he got worried or upset his pain was worse. He was not sure how to avoid the upset that caused it, or how to reduce his worry when it did happen.

He started doing relaxation classes and became more and more skilled at noticing very early signs of upset. At first he thought the earliest sign was a knotted stomach and sweaty palms. As he got better at relaxing so he got better at noticing the slight tenseness in his jaw and a quickening of his heart beat. This seemed to be an even earlier sign. Once he was good at seeing these earliest signs of tension he became better at dealing with the things that upset him, either avoiding them or learning to feel calmer about them.

Once you have got to the stage where you are using relaxation almost automatically, you will get better at noticing the early signs of tension. The earlier you can apply your relaxation technique, the less tension there is to reduce.

At first these exercises will feel rather self-conscious and deliberate, but they are worth the effort, because they will soon come more naturally and be more automatic. Remember the object of all this work is to have a relaxed response ready for normal situations like sitting on the bus or shopping. There is no doubt it feels better to be relaxed than to be tense.

By now you will have a good idea of what makes you tense, and you will be better at reducing it. This should be helping some of your pain, but you will have noticed many daily activities still give you pain. The next part of the programme is the most crucial. It expects you to put together all the knowledge you have gathered so far and redesign a more rewarding daily life.

5. Making changes: Activity

▶ What has pain stopped you doing?
▶ Knowing when to stop
▶ Recording your activities
▶ Setting targets
▶ Trial and error
▶ Accepting your limits

It is now time to take stock and see how your pain affects your everyday life in practice. Sit down quietly for a couple of hours when you know you will not be interrupted and make four lists in answer to the following questions:

1. What have I given up doing
    since I have had so much pain **?**

2. What things would I
    like to be able to do again **?**

3. What new things would I
    like to be doing in the future **?**

4. What are the reasons for
    not doing as much as I used to **?**

The last question is more difficult. It requires some soul-searching because you need to be able to distinguish between those activities which you don't do because of the pain, and those you are actually no longer able to do physically.

When you try to answer this question it may help to go through a number of smaller questions. For example:

▶ Is it only the pain
   which stops me doing things **?**

▶ Am I frightened
   that I'll damage myself **?**

▶ Am I not doing things or going
   out because I have lost my confidence **?**

▶ Have I lost the will
   or energy to do things **?**

▶ Is this loss of interest only because of the pain, or are
   there other things in my life
   which are bringing me down **?**

▶ Do I sometimes use the pain as an excuse not to do
   something that I was never
   very keen on doing anyway **?**

▶ Are there
   opportunities to do any more **?**

▶ Is it because I can't think what to do or is it because there
   is nowhere to go,
   nobody to go with **?**

Should I stop when it hurts?

Amongst our pain clinic patients one of the main reasons for
no longer living a full and interesting life is that activity brings
on the pain or makes existing pain much worse. This is
understandable to some extent because nobody feels like
doing much when they are in pain, and they often ask 'Should
I stop when it hurts?'

As a general rule if you have already been checked
thoroughly by a doctor whom you trust and with whom you
are able to discuss your intentions, this will guide you. You
can then avoid things she or he thinks won't help. If you
want to try your programme alone then you should still note
down any major changes in pain or sensations that concern
you. You can choose to discuss these with the doctor later,
and check that you are not damaging yourself.

Giving in to pain means doing less and less, gradually becoming less inclined to go out, meet friends, or do many of the things you used to do.

Cancelling an evening out or not bothering to phone a friend for a chat is OK for those who only get the occasional headache or period pain. But for those who have frequent or permanent pain this response is dangerous.

The loss of a spontaneous and active lifestyle is one of the main problems for people in pain; it gets very depressing and lonely. With this comes a feeling of hopelessness and isolation. The pain becomes more prominent as there is less to do and daily life becomes more and more restricted. For some people this feeling goes on for years, and mobility is reduced to a few steps. They continue to harbour resentment and wait for a cure.

This attitude has to go. It makes you more disabled than you need be and stops you getting on with yourlife.

Recording your activity

Is it really the pain that is stopping you doing things?

This week's recording will help you examine to what extent your activity is restricted because you fear that it will hurt. This sort of fear can be as crippling as the pain itself. But reducing activity is not necessarily the most sensible way of coping. Rather than just cutting down activity, it is worth getting to understand more about the way different types of activity affect your pain. That way you can find ways round your pain, and still stay active.

The recording exercise in Chapter 3 (page 22) may have given you a reasonable idea of the sort of physical activity that does not suit you. You may already know this, but it should help to make a note of what you did prior to a period of more severe pain, since sometimes the effect can be quite delayed.

Peter discovered that his back pain was very much worse three days after he had been pinning up children's pictures at the primary school where he taught. The pain did not start immediately, but he noticed his back stiffening up as he sat relaxing in the evening. He found himself so stiff and sore the next day that he had to remain in bed. Close monitoring over a few weeks showed him that this stretching and pushing movement tended to be the culprit. He swopped an extra playground duty with his colleague who pinned up his class's pictures for him. By doing this he reduced one of the major sources of his bad pain.

If, in your case, it seems that almost anything you do causes pain, then you will need to start by keeping a regular daily record of activity. Here is an example of an activity record noting pain level and activity every two hours.

Activity record sheet

Day/time	Pain rating (0–5)	What I have been doing during the last two hours
8am	0	Asleep
10am	1	Driving / Shopping
Noon	3	Housework / Cooking
2pm	0	Resting

What have I learnt in week four?

Gathering this information over seven days should help you understand more about the relationship between your activity and your pain. You will notice how some effects may only be apparent a few hours later, and that some activities are more likely to be followed by higher levels of pain than others. By learning about your activity in this way you will be in a better position to control your pain, because you will be much more aware of those activities which need to be avoided or undertaken with care. Some people find some activities that cause pain don't have to be dropped completely – they can pace them out better, resting more between activities, or maybe doing loosening up exercises before starting.

Olive found a number of activities were problematic, such as hoovering or driving, but many others were not, for example watching TV or cooking. Her record for one day is shown here.

Olive's activity diary

Day/time Wed.	Pain rating	Tension rating	What I have been doing during last two hours
8 - 10	4	3	Hoovering and housework.
10 - 12	3/4	2	Resting.
12 - 2	3	1	Walking round the shops.
2 - 4	2	1	Picking kids up from school.
4 - 6	2	0	Having tea, watching T.V.
6 - 8	4	3	Chatting to relatives.

Olive also recorded her *TENSION* level because she realized that for her even the thought of some activity produced tension and gave her more pain.

It will be important when you begin to increase your activities to keep a careful check on your tension in case it is this and not the pain which is making matters worse and stopping you from doing things. Perhaps if you think this is important in your case, you could include a tension column yourself in your activity record. To help you, here are seven activity record diary pages which you can complete yourself.

45

Activity record diary

Day/time	Pain rating	Tension rating	What I have been doing during last two hours

Day/time	Pain rating	Tension rating	What I have been doing during last two hours

Day/time	Pain rating	Tension rating	What I have been doing during last two hours

Day/time	Pain rating	Tension rating	What I have been doing during last two hours

Day/time	Pain rating	Tension rating	What I have been doing during last two hours

Day/time	Pain rating	Tension rating	What I have been doing during last two hours

Day/time	Pain rating	Tension rating	What I have been doing during last two hours

Making changes

Having got some idea of what activities you want to try, and knowing which ones you can do in comfort, you are in a strong position to increase your activities. Your first step will be to plan an activity programme.

Setting yourself targets

Select a series of activity targets to be completed each day. These can be as small or as large as you like, depending on what you can manage.

The word 'programme' implies a systematic and gradual approach. You should select targets or activities and build them up at a pace which suits you. You will have to choose your own pace so you feel confident, and do not unduly increase your pain.

The programme should start with activities that cause you least pain. You should start by doing them at a time you are most likely to succeed. For example, you may have learned that your pain has a distinct pattern over the day, so you will need to specify times for doing certain things. (If you loosen up as the day goes on, take your walk in the afternoon or evening.)

The targets need to be specified very clearly for you to be able to measure success, and to note whether you have gone too quickly, should you hurt a lot afterwards.

The following list shows a very wide range of targets chosen by people with greatly varying degrees of disability.

▶ Walking 10/20/30 steps every day.
▶ Walking for 5/10/15-60 minutes evey day.
▶ Walking to the end of the drive/road/town.
▶ Gardening for 5/10/60 minutes.
▶ Making a coffee/gravy.
▶ Preparing the potatoes for supper.
▶ Cooking a meal.
▶ Playing a game of cards, draughts, darts, bowls, each day.

Setting personal targets

Write down your own personal targets for tomorrow:

_____

_____

_____

_____

Specify targets clearly for each day, then after your have tried them you can write down your pain rating and your comments. Here is an example of a completed target diary for one week.

Target diary

Day	Target	Pain	Comments
Mon	Walk 5 mins	4	Possibly too fast; take it slower.
Tues	Walk 5 mins	3	Better when slower.
Wed	Walk 5 mins	3	Not Bad!
Thurs	Walk 5 mins	1	Going well; try 10 mins tomorrow.
Fri	Walk 10 mins	3	Better than I expected tired; maybe I went too fast.
Sat	Walk 10 mins	3	Take it slower!
Sun	Walk 10 mins	2	Took longer, but worth it.

49

Trial and error

You will find that this trial and error period will provide valuable information on what exercise you can build on, and what feels worse and what better. You cannot ignore the pain nor can you ignore the fact that your physical abilities may be restricted. Indeed if you do ignore these then you risk forcing yourself beyond your limits and you will suffer more pain as a result. Rushing into vigorous exercise is clearly not advised; if you do hurt a lot after your target session this means you have probably overdone it. A well-designed programme is one where the new activity is paced so that it can be built up slowly without too much increase in pain. Remember that if you have been doing very little it will hurt even more when you start trying to move again.

This advice may sound a little confusing. It's going to hurt a little as you try new things and you try to get back to a more active life. This is to be expected. But if you notice any major changes in the quality of your pain, or very long-lasting or severe pain, this will tell you you've either done too much, or you have misjudged the sort of things to try. Unfortunately, changes are likely to give some increase in pain – but it will be worth it in the longer term.

> *John was a bit hesitant about taking up swimming again. He started gently, but, even so, was quite stiff for the rest of the day. After two or three weeks of regular sessions he found he was more supple, and was getting some strength back into his legs.*
>
> *Although he felt stiffer immediately after the exercise he was delighted to find his general fitness building up over the long-term. He really felt he had turned the corner.*

Green – Amber – Red

After a couple of weeks trying to set targets and pace yourself you should have a pretty good idea of which activities are no problem, which are alright in moderation and which are definitely to be avoided. We can call these *GREEN, AMBER* and *RED* activities respectively. Just to check that you are getting the hang of this fill in the chart below to identify your *GREEN, AMBER* and *RED* activities. This will act as a

50

reminder, so that if you overdo things or if you find yourself making excuses for doing very little you will know who to blame!

GREEN (Safe activities)	AMBER (Take it steady)	RED (To be avoided)

The see-saw

It is particularly important to take things at a steady pace and to maintain a calm and positive attitude. There will often be a tendency to 'Catastrophize' when you become either very impatient with the pain or give in to it completely. If you catastrophize you will do badly and make the worst of your pain because you will find yourself on a see-saw – some days overdoing things and others doing almost nothing. It will feel as if you are being thrown from one end of the see-saw to the other: forever going up and down but never quite getting it right.

Think about some of the days you have had recently when you felt like this. Try and remember what you were doing on those days and say at which end of the all-or-nothing see-saw these activities belong. Write them down at the appropriate end of the see-saw in the diagram on page 52 and see whether you tend to be an 'Overdoer', an 'Underdoer' or whether you seem to career between the two.

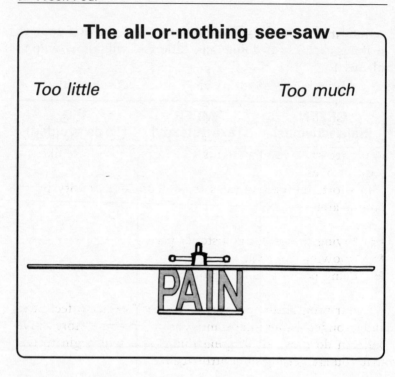

The all-or-nothing see-saw

Too little *Too much*

We can always see the difference between a positive and a negative approach in our patients. Those who think positively do much better than those who think there is little they can do to control their life. Here are some typical statements demonstrating the difference between a positive and a negative attitude to the problem.

Positive statements	*Negative statements*
'I am gradually going to get on top of this problem.'	'Why me? It's not fair. I've always taken good care of my health.'
'I am coping well, all things considered.'	'What's the point? Taking exercise doesn't get rid of the pain.'
'I know I can manage if I keep going at a steady pace.'	'I'd better not go. I'll never manage and I'll be a nuisance.'

Look back at the things you have recorded in the see-saw exercise and try to recollect which sort of statement was likely to have been going through your mind at the time. You are likely to find that during activities or on days near either end of the see-saw your thoughts will be similar to the list of negative statements. On days when you feel good and keep going at a steady and manageable pace (that is, in the middle of the see-saw) your thoughts and attitude are more like the positive ones.

In short, the prerequisites for a successful activity programme are:

▶ Trying things out at a steady pace.
▶ Knowing your limits.
▶ Being positive and keeping calm.

As your programme progresses you will begin to feel fitter and stronger. More importantly, as you become more active and can do more challenging things you will begin to feel that you are getting in control again.

Accepting your limits

This chapter has described how you can extend the limits of your physical activity. For some there will always be severe limitations which mean having to accept being 'disabled'. There can be an enormous sense of grief at the loss of full health. This is possibly something only the sufferer can properly appreciate.

However, the feats of many very disabled people are testimony to the fact that being disabled physically does not mean being totally disabled as a human being. Yet we often see people who have been in pain for a long time, and they have gradually become disabled in social, emotional and intellectual terms as well. Accepting that your body is not as good as it used to be is a hard and lonely lesson, but one which has to be addressed, so that you are then free to build a future.

If you are disabled you will need to look for ways to manage in spite of this. It may involve changing some of the essential everyday chores to suit your problem (for example bed making, hoovering, lifting, typing). In addition, you may need to change your environment (for example seating, heating, rails, bed height). The local community occupational therapist in your social services department and the disabled living centres are worth contacting for help in this area (see *Addresses of Useful Organizations*).

Coping despite your disability may also involve looking for new hobbies and interests in the way that Ruth has. She is a 63-year-old retired teacher who has developed a good understanding of what she has to avoid. She adjusted her lifestyle to suit her disability and continues to live a rich and fulfilling life.

> '*I have to walk more slowly now, and I stopped going out with the rambling club, although walking on flat ground is one of the things I still do to ease my backache. Sitting and lying are the worst culprits. I go shopping very frequently to avoid carrying too much at one go, and I always get my neighbour to help with heavy jobs like turning matresses. I help her in return by doing errands on my many journeys to the shops! I have just taken up a daytime course in local history which I really enjoy. It's full of interesting characters who have lived in the area all their lives. They don't seem to mind me getting up to stretch my legs every few minutes.*'

Suddenly finding that you are prevented from doing things because of physical disability can leave gaps in your life which you may feel can never be filled. Remember, you can still get the most out of your social and intellectual abilities, however physically restricted you may have become. Filling the gaps will need imagination and tenacity but it is possible if you are determined. You may even be surprised as you discover bits of yourself you never knew you had as you try out new things.

6. Getting services to work for you

▶ Getting information
▶ Asking the right questions
▶ What treatments are available?
▶ Assessing costs and benefits

So many people in pain seem unhappy or disappointed with the services they have received. Some people feel let down by the doctors who failed to cure them, others feel they are left to deal with long-term pain all on their own. The most common complaint from people who have been in pain for many years is the difficulty they have in getting clear information on their problems.

In an ideal world doctors would share what they know with their patients, deal with them all cheerfully and honestly, and pain sufferers would all be cured. Of course, the truth is that pain is something of a puzzle both to the professionals and to the sufferer. Because of the limits of knowledge many people feel let down.

Doctors are human like the rest of us, and do, on occasions, fail to answer questions properly and get disappointed with themselves and their technology when they fail to help patients. Patients notice doctors starting off so optimistically, but their disappointment and frustration becomes evident as the patient fails to get better.

This chapter is designed to help pain sufferers get the best out of health services. The issues covered here are based on a national survey of back pain sufferers. From this survey we know that sufferers want more information, more humane care, and more access to a wider variety of treatments, both traditional medical and complementary or alternative treatments.

Getting information

Most sufferers want more information. They want to know about the cause of their problem, what is wrong, whether they are likely to get any worse and guidance on how to cope better.

Hospital outpatient visits can be fraught with difficulties. One patient told us what a disappointment her visits to the hospital usually were. She was still not clear what was wrong with her back and legs, and she wanted to know whether it was going to get worse. Unfortunately, she had a long and uncomfortable journey to the hospital, and she usually had to wait around, so by the time her turn came she had forgotten all the questions she wanted to ask. She put a brave face on it at the time, but when she got home she just broke down and cried.

This is a familiar story, but there are ways round it. You could take a close relative or friend along with you next time. They will be less anxious, and should remember more than you about the clinic visits, and the two of you can discuss it later.

Another way round this problem is to prepare a list of questions in advance of going to the doctor. Take care in choosing these questions as the way in which you ask questions can determine how much you find out.

There is certainly a skill to preparing your questions briefly and succinctly, and if you jot them down on a piece of paper leave enough space to put in a reply; then you can note down what the doctor says at the time, and can mull over it later.

It may be that the doctor you see is not very keen to answer some of the questions because he simply doesn't know the answer.

Many of us put doctors up on a pedestal, and expect them to be the expert who knows everything. Not all doctors are like that, but we have all met some doctors who behave as if they are on a pedestal. Most people (and that includes doctors) are reasonable and want to share information that might help you. But the medical answers will very rarely be framed in the definite 'clear cut' way you probably want.

What sort of questions to ask

Doctors are very unwilling to say you will definitely get better or definitely get worse. They work in probabilities, and are more prepared to give you some kind of 'likelihood' answer rather than a black or white one.

PATIENT: *Am I going to get better?*
DOCTOR: *I would say your chances of getting better are pretty small.*
PATIENT: *How small?*
DOCTOR: *Probably less than 1 in 20 people I have seen with your problem got any better.*

It is just as tricky asking about the pain.

PATIENT: *Will the pain get worse?*
DOCTOR: *It may get worse, or then again you may be lucky.*

But if you ask him about probabilities, you may get a clearer answer.

PATIENT: *Is it possible to tell me if my pain is likely to get any worse or likely to get any better?*
DOCTOR: *I'm afraid it's more likely to get worse.*

You might also try other probability questions.

PATIENT: *Is there any treatment that might help with my sort of problem?*
PATIENT: *Is it likely that the drug I am taking is going to have side-effects in the long-term?*

The doctor will very rarely give you a definite yes or no, and will prefer to answer questions put this way. It is less clear-cut for you, but more likely to get you an answer!

Getting answers

The following section suggests the way to approach medical practitioners to get good, clear advice. You may have tried this already and been unsuccessful, but don't give up. It may be that you asked difficult or impossible questions, or you may have been told something you didn't want to hear. Try the following:

1. Go to a health professional that you trust.

2. Work out your questions at home before you go to the clinic. You are much more likely to feel relaxed and think systematically and clearly at home. If you leave it too late you will feel anxious or on edge and you will leave out the important questions.

    Anxiety has a dramatic and negative effect on concentration and memory, so make it easier for yourself and prepare beforehand. You can bring your written notes home later to ponder over and discuss with your family and friends.

3. Don't be frightened to ask questions. Take a list of written questions, and even give the doctor a copy before you start. Take a note pad to write down the answers. Take someone along with you, your partner, friend or daughter, so that they can listen as well. They will probably remember more than you.

4. Take your monitoring forms along with you, and summarize them clearly for the doctor.

5. Always ask the doctor to explain any words you don't understand.

Self-monitoring

The information you choose to take with you will mainly depend on the questions you want answered at that particular visit.

Your self-monitoring will have helped you make some sense of your pattern of pain, and the way certain activities are affecting it. You will also note whether you are taking pills at the right times. Your monitoring may also show useful information that you don't necessarily understand, but it may help your doctor to make a more accurate diagnosis. For instance, the time of day the pain or stiffness is worse, or the way certain pills affect your pain can all help diagnosis, so giving information to the doctor on your activity and when you are taking your pills and the effect these have on you can be worthwhile.

In the back of your mind you may have the idea that there is something very seriously wrong with you. Now is the time to check it. An example of a summary sheet that you could take to the doctor is included at the end of this chapter. Meanwhile here are some suggestions for questions to ask your doctor.

Suggested questions

▶ Can you tell me the name for what is wrong with me?

▶ How do you think it started?

▶ Why does it hurt all the way down my left leg?

▶ Is it likely to get better if I stop work as an office cleaner?

▶ Is there an operation that is likely to help me?

▶ Is it likely to get worse if I have another baby?

▶ Is it likely to get better if I go jogging?

▶ Is it likely to get better if I go to bed for a week?

What treatments are available?

In our own survey doctors were not found to be terribly helpful in answering questions clearly on the wide range of treatments available. They are often not prepared to recommend types of complementary or alternative treatments (for example osteopathy, reflexology, Alexander technique), even though the people we asked had often found these methods very helpful. Perhaps this is not so surprising since doctors have no control over these forms of treatment or their practitioners, and they don't feel that they can be responsible even for giving advice on them.

For these reasons we have included a list of useful addresses at the back of the book so you can seek out this information for yourself. As far as possible we have included chartered or registered and well-respected groups, but you really do need to check them out for yourself. National self-help groups, like the Back Pain Association, have local branches, and these are good places to contact people who have used local practitioners and can give informed word-of-mouth recommendations.

Can I get treatment at a pain relief clinic?

Generally, you will need to be referred by your own GP or hospital consultant to be seen in a pain relief clinic. If your own GP doesn't want to refer you to one you can try ringing the clinic directly to see if they can advise you on what to do. In Britain these clinics are run mainly by anaesthetists, and the major treatments are medical and use invasive methods. These are methods which interfere with the body's process (for example pills), or involve some invasion of the body (such as operations and injections). But this is not always the case, and some clinics will have a slightly broader approach (for example acupuncture, yoga, hypnosis). Again, the pain relief clinic secretary may be able to answer your questions on what they offer.

In the list of useful addresses we have included the Intractable Pain Society, the organization concerned with pain relief. They can send out lists of local pain relief clinics.

Assessing the costs and benefits of treatment

It is sometimes difficult to decide whether to try a treatment. A useful way to view this decision is to compare the costs and benefits.

While some methods are quite effective, they may give too high a 'cost' to the sufferer. So on balance the sufferer may decide that the 'cost' of taking, say, pain killers is higher than the 'benefit' of getting rid of the pain. In our survey we found that although some medical treatments were found to be quite effective, people were not always very happy with their side-effects.

> *Clive was a manual worker. He'd had back pain for many years, and although his spinal fusion took most of his original pain away, he was unable to return to work because of difficulty with moving and bending. He found it so restricting he sometimes wished the operation had not been done.*

What about side-effects?

Our survey also revealed that many people found that pills helped the pain, but they didn't like the side-effects like feeling sleepy, and they regretted being dependent on pills. Many were frightened of the possible long-term effects. Also, taking certain pills meant restricting alcohol, or watching particular foods or even having to take extra pills to deal with the side-effects of the pain killers. So very often, although the pills were rated as being quite effective, some people found that they preferred to deal even with the high levels of pain they were getting without pills, because the side-effects were so unacceptable.

> *Bob, the electronic engineer who felt trapped and miserable, found that strong pain killers helped the pain. Unfortunately, he had to take more than the prescribed dose to touch the pain, and felt hungover and dreadful for a couple of days afterwards. He decided that the 'cost' was too high for the 'benefit' of getting rid of the pain just to get one good night's sleep.*

Making your decision

It is up to you to weigh up whether you wish to go ahead with any particular treatment, deciding whether it seems very costly for the benefits of effective pain control. If the costs are high, the benefits have to be very high too. If the costs are low (as with non-invasive methods like a nerve stimulator) then the benefits can be low.

Only you can assess costs and benefits and make decisions on any treatments offered. Doctors may not see 'success' in quite the way that you do. Taking the pain away, although clearly important, is not the only consideration, particularly with invasive methods. It is you that will have to live with any additional 'costs' or side-effects of the treatment you try. You don't have to have a treatment just because it is offered. If in doubt, make sure the doctor answers each of your questions on the likely costs of the treatments.

What are my pills for?

	Name of pill	Colour	What are they for?	What time of day should I take them?
1				
2				
3				
4				
5				

Getting information: summary sheet

Here is an example of a summary sheet that you could take to the clinic to get clear answers.

Don't be afraid to modify it to suit your own needs!

NAME _____

DOCTOR'S NAME _____

CLINIC _____ DATE _____

What do you think is wrong with me? _____

What is likely to have started it off? _____

Do you think it is likely to get worse/better/stay the same?

How quickly is that likely to happen? _____

What can I do that might help the pain (e.g. exercise, lose weight)? _____

Are there any activities I could do that might help it?

_____

What should I try to avoid? _____

What other treatments are likely to help this sort of problem?

_____

What are likely to be the side-effects of these treatments?

_____

What complementary treatments would you firmly advise me against? _____

Why? _____

What alternative treatments do you think are likely to help this kind of problem? _____

Is my pain likely to get worse if I get pregnant again? / I go back to work? / I take up swimming? _____

7. Pain: some puzzles and possible answers

▶ What is pain?
▶ What affects the way we feel pain?
▶ Gate Theory
▶ Relaxation
▶ Imagery
▶ Hypnosis
▶ Biofeedback
▶ Operant techniques

This chapter is included for those who are intrigued about their pain and want to know a bit more about new ways of helping people with pain. Indeed, understanding some of the theoretical background may make it easier to see why the most unexpected remedies sometimes work, and particularly why self-help is now seen as important.

What is pain?

The most basic fact to start from is that pain is not simply a message, like a phone call, sent to your brain to tell you something is wrong with your body. Pain is more complex than that, and although we usually hurt when we are injured, a pain message sent to your brain can get changed or waylaid by all sorts of psychological processes.

Does pain have any purpose?

Pain certainly serves a useful purpose when you are injured. It makes you stop in your tracks, so you take avoiding action.

You take your hand out of the flame, or remove the paving stone from your foot. Here it has a 'survival' value.

But if you think back more carefully to the last few times you were injured you will notice that on some occasions an injury can hurt very badly, and on others it hardly hurts at all. Pain is something of a puzzle, and the way we experience it differently at different times is not fully understood. When you have had pain well beyond normal healing time it is difficult to see what sort of survival value this can possibly have. It is these sorts of puzzles that we are really interested in, and it is these real-life observations that have formed the basis of current theories of what pain is all about.

What affects the way we experience pain?

The puzzles which we list now have intrigued scientists studying pain. They make researchers look for some more comprehensive explanations that take psychological factors into account.

Phantom limb pain. Why, for instance, do some people feel pain in their foot after their leg has been amputated? If we are simply dealing with a telegraph system, where is the message coming from, when there is no foot? Why does it feel as if there is still a complete leg when the foot is not there?

This obsevation suggests that our brain is so powerful that it can even create a feeling of the foot still being there, in spite of the sufferer knowing perfectly well that the leg has been amputated.

Mind over-riding pain. It also seems that the brain plays an important part in deciding whether to let a pain message through, because on some occasions it has been noticed that people with quite severe injuries do not notice any pain. For instance, many of you will have read of, or even seen, people being quite seriously injured half-way through an important football or rugby match, but they only seem to notice the pain when the game is finished. They are amazed to find they have broken bones, and that the pain is suddenly quite excruciating.

66

Again, this suggests that the brain has a very powerful influence on the pain message.

Personal differences. Why is it that two people with very similar injuries or infections often feel it very differently? One seems to suffer very badly, while the other hardly seems to notice it at all. You may have noticed some of your friends tolerate pain very badly and others have a very stoical attitude and cope with it well. People are clearly different in the way they react to pain.

These differences between individuals are difficult to explain. They are probably due to physical, psychological and social differences between people. For example, since the nervous system itself does not react in the same way in everybody, it could be that the frequency and intensity of pain messages vary across people. We know from studies of children in pain that they are taught how to react by their parents and that they copy their parents' behaviour when they are ill or in pain. Not only do we learn from the family how to respond to pain but our culture expects us to respond in certain ways. Some cultures expect loud wailing whilst others expect a stiff upper lip. Likewise, everyday social situations influence the way we feel pain and our reactions to it.

Painwatching. You may also have noticed that when you sit and think about your pain and attend to it very carefully then it hurts more. Similarly, if you switch your mind away from the pain you notice it less. So when you are with some of your good friends having a laugh and a joke, you are very easily distracted and don't notice the pain quite so much.

We are not suggesting that the pain goes away when you are absorbed in something interesting, but it does seem that you notice it less.

Tension. Many people have commented that when they get tense and upset that's when their pain gets worse. Of course pain itself makes us more tense. This is a bit of a trap, because tension itself can make you hurt more, which may make you more tense.

Mood. If you are feeling rushed or under pressure your pain is likely to become worse. It has also been noticed that people with long-term pain can get very depressed. This is not so surprising if people are feeling helpless and trapped by it, but research also shows us that if we can find some way to reduce the pain then the depression lifts. This suggests that, for some people, pain causes depression. But depression has two faces. Although it is often caused by pain, being depressed can also make you experience more pain.

The meaning of pain. One further piece of evidence that is often quoted by scientists came from an astute piece of observation many years ago.

Soldiers injured badly in the Boer War very rarely asked for pain killers. When they were compared with civilians who had had similar injuries, but were not fighting in a war, it was noticed that the soldiers asked for pain killers far less often than the civilians. Although they both had the same sort of injuries it seemed that the meaning of the injury was significant. The soldiers found their pain was less important, because for them their injury had advantages: it was a 'ticket home'. The civilians were probably very frightened and worried about what was going to happen to them, and since surgery was very hazardous in those days, they saw no great advantage in having pain.

All these examples demonstrate the importance of mind over matter. As observations and evidence they certainly show that the mind has a big effect on how much our pain hurts, and how much we attend to it. They demonstrate how we can over-ride, exaggerate or even delay noticing pain messages.

Can gate theory answer these puzzles?

Gate Control Theory has been one of the most significant recent developments in our understanding of pain. Until recently it was thought that we hurt because there was some injury to the body. The greater the damage, the greater the pain we would feel. Gate Control Theory tries to explain the observations noted above, which suggest that pain is not such a simple matter.

It is a well-named theory, using the idea of a gate which can open to allow pain messages through, or can shut to stop messages. For example, when we are tense the gate will tend to open more, if we are calm and relaxed it will tend to shut. This begins to explain why sometimes we hurt, and at other times we don't – even when the cause stays the same.

If we look carefully at things that open and shut this gate then it can give us ideas on how to try to shut the gate more often. This can become the basis for your own programme, which aims to reduce the pain you feel.

What makes the gate open?

Pain seems to get worse when there is:

▶ *Physical damage.* The size and type of damage can influence the amount of pain which is felt, and the way it feels. For instance, shingles pain will feel very different from scar pain as it originates from very different causes.

▶ *Low activity.* You will notice the pain when you are doing less because activity has a distracting effect. So you will cause yourself more problems if your activity reduces a lot, because you are then likely to notice the pain more.

▶ *Depression/helplessness.* People who feel a lot of pain will tend to do less and get out of the swing of things. As you do less so the positives in life also get fewer, and there is less opportunity to get enjoyment out of things. Many people describe trapped and helpless feelings, and their lower mood will make the pain worse.

▶ *Anger.* We have often seen people angry with medical services. They expect to be cured, and get disappointed if they are not: they feel let down and annoyed. They may also be angry at their disability, asking 'Why me?' and feel it's unfair that they've been singled out.

69

▶ *Stress/tension*. There are two ways tension makes pain worse. Pain in itself can cause tension, because it is natural to tense up to try to stop yourself hurting more. And if you allow yourself to get very tense, then this opens the gate, and you will feel more pain.

▶ *Painwatching*. If you attend more to the pain you will notice it more. Attending to it opens the gate.

▶ *Fear about what the pain is*. Getting accurate information about your pain is nearly always much less frightening than your secret worries about what is causing your pain. Many people secretly worry there is something very seriously wrong, and this can build up and lead to tension and anxiety which will open the gate to pain.

What makes the gate close?

These seem to help close the gate and reduce the pain:

▶ *Pain killers* and some antidepressants will make you notice the pain less.

▶ *Counter-stimulation*. Some of you will have had heat treatment or massage or even cold compresses which can help to spread the effect of the pain and close the gate at spinal level.

▶ *Keeping busy*, keeping attention off the pain. If you can keep busy and switch your attention away from it you will help close the gate.

▶ *Being relaxed*. Reducing your anxiety and learning to relax can all help reduce the pain messages getting through.

▶ *Setting realistic targets for your life*. This is essential so you can make the best of things. You can reduce helplessness and tension by achieving small goals which you set for yourself and feel are rewarding. Taking this positive attitude to life will help, because you are beginning to take control.

Pain = mind + body!

It is these factors that we have in mind when we say that pain is partly psychological and partly physical, and that you can reduce the amount of pain you feel. So, for example, even if you have a physical problem like arthritis you can still get a better deal out of it if you are feeling relaxed and happy. This is because the gate is more shut than when you are feeling hopeless, dissatisfied or worried.

In summary, the pain we feel seems to be influenced by numerous factors. Some of these have to do with the physical state of our body and the amount of damage that is suffered. Other factors have more to do with our feelings, our thoughts and our state of mind.

It is these characteristics that we have emphasized throughout this book because these are things you can alter and do something about.

What treatments are based on the psychological research?

Because the programme described throughout this book is based on self-help methods, these will not be repeated here. The information included here is intended to add to your knowledge. You will notice that often the principles are similar to those you are now using in the programme you have designed for yourself. We have concentrated on describing treatments you are most likely to hear mentioned or be offered.

These are some of the particular psychological techniques that can help.

Relaxation

Relaxation has been found to be very useful with pain problems for three reasons which you may recognize:

1. Pain is stressful and makes you tense.

2. Pain makes you 'guard' to protect your body from more pain.

3. A high level of tension makes the pain feel worse.

In well-designed studies relaxation comes out as a useful treatment for the widest variety of pain problems.

▶   The act of learning relaxation seems to help you identify the effects of tension in these three different ways.
▶   So relaxation can help you gain extra feelings of control, and as tension reduces, so it can also reduce your pain.
▶   Relaxation also reduces blood pressure, muscle tension and it increases blood flow to the fingers and toes.

James is 40 years old. He had a bad whiplash injury in a road traffic accident five years ago and has to wear a surgical collar most of the time. He always seemed to have a stiff neck and shoulders, and a headache like a tight band round his head.
Relaxation helped him to stop 'guarding' and the extra problems of headache and muscle stiffness seemed much better.

The exercises given in Chapter 4 are the ones clinics usually start with. Some of you may have been given a tape to learn from. It is always harder to learn such a new skill on your own, and some programmes may even take up to ten sessions teaching these techniques. So it will not be easy to learn from a book, but it's a start, and there may well be local sessions you can attend, to back-up your own efforts.

Guided imagery

Because people in pain know that switching attention from the pain helps them notice it less, the professionals have developed methods to help sufferers attention-switch, or reinterpret the particular sensation.

> *Gwen had always had bad legs and at last was having her varicose veins done just after she had retired. The healing was slow, leaving a very painful scar, even after the surgeon had reoperated to try to release any trapped nerves in the scar tissue.*
>
> *There were two pains. A dull ache, with her all the time, and a stabbing pain which came occasionally, without any warning. When she monitored carefully, she found out that the dull pain got worse with tension – but the stabbing pain seemed impossible to control. She found it frighteningly powerful.*
>
> *Because the stabbing pain was so frightening, and there seemed little she could do to shift or reduce it, we discussed the idea of using her thoughts to make the pain seem different and less fearful. She became skilled in deep relaxation and clever at imagining the sudden pain as a heavy or massage-like pressure, and she found this took some of the fear out of it, particularly as she felt more in control.*

Another method might have been for her to learn to switch attention away from the site of pain, or to use another form of guided imagery, by building up a scene in her mind (for example in a deep wood, by a river, by the sea, in a friendly room) and imagining herself there. This would take her right out of the present and into a newly-created, pain-free place.

It is the reinterpretation method described first that seems to work best. Any of these methods should help, but sometimes it is easier to get the effect using the same methods, but with a therapist to guide you and lead your thoughts.

Hypnosis

Hypnosis is a valuable tool for pain management, but needs skilled application. Once deeply induced to a trance-like state, people can show amazing control over their pain.

Some phantom-limb patients use hypnosis to shift the sharp sensation they feel in their stump, down the phantom leg, and out at the end.

Moving the pain around the body, and creating a new, controllable pain in another part of your body can also help you switch attention away from the site of pain.

One man who came to see us had injured his left arm in an industrial accident. He worked out some clever and original ways of dealing with his nine identified pains in this arm, but had difficulty in getting rid of a gnawing pain in this thumb that occasionally kept him awake at night, and seemed worse in cold weather.

He was trained in self-hypnosis and he practised it at home. He used a technique of creating pain in his good, right arm. He imagined he was clutching onto the hand rail of a flight of stairs with his good hand, but clutching it so tightly that it hurt. This new sensation grabbed all his attention, and the original left arm pain was much reduced. He also felt more in control.

You may well be tempted to go to a local hypnotist – but it is wise to check, by local recommendations, whether they are good. If this is not possible, check with the two major professional bodies, The British Society of Medical and Dental Hypnotists or the British Society of Hypnotherapists (see *Addresses of Useful Organizations*). Hypnosis is available on the NHS in some pain relief clinics or psychology departments. (Check details with your own doctor.)

Biofeedback

You may have seen relaxometers advertised in popular magazines. Small electronic devices, with little pads (electrodes) you place on your skin, they are designed to help you relax better. These devices generally focus on muscle tension, sweating, heart rate or temperature. You will have noticed that all these are signs of tension, so if you can learn to control any one of these responses better, your general tension should reduce.

The machines are designed to take one particular measure of your tension. When you place the electrodes or contacts on yourself, the machine will amplify and electronically measure the response your body gives. You may see a dial or a series of lights, or hear a tone rising and falling with the changing messages your body gives the machine. This machine is providing feedback to you on how well you are relaxing. In a series of practice sessions you will begin to learn to reduce these tense responses by learning to keep the tone down or the lights off. So, biofeedback can help you generally relax better.

The best way to use biofeedback is in teaching yourself to control those particular responses that may be giving you pain, such as tension headache (by reducing muscle tension). You may have Reynaud's Disease (a problem with circulation, particularly in fingers and toes), which can be helped by learning to keep the temperature in your extremities to a steady and higher level.

Biofeedback has been particularly useful for phantom limb pain; jaw pain; tension headache and Reynaud's Disease.

Operant programmes

Operant programmes are based on theories of learning which predict that behaviour that is rewarded will occur more often. Inpatient operant programmes have become popular in the USA to help people who have become very inactive. They are put into a strict, highly controlled regime which encourages them to steadily build up a more active life. These major goals are broken down into small steps, and every achievement, however small, is reinforced.

These intensive inpatient programmes seem better suited to the American insurance-based health system and the problems of drug dependency often found amongst American pain sufferers. There are just a handful of operant programmes in Britain. They are designed primarily to help two sorts of people: those who have difficulty motivating themselves to get going through a self-management programme like the one described in this book; and those who have a family who encourage them in their passive and disabled role.

We hope that this chapter has clarified some of the theoretical issues involved in pain management. If you want more information, the next section, *Addresses of Useful Organizations,* gives contact addresses for a variety of organizations and professional bodies.

Addresses of Useful Organizations

Rights

Organizations to contact for advice on the legal, statutory and discretionary rights of disabled people.

Arthritis and Rheumatism Council
41 Eagle Street
London
WC1R 4AR
Tel: 01 405 8572

Association of Disabled
   Professionals
The Stables
73 Pound Road
Banstead
Surrey
SM7 2HU
Tel: 073 73 52366

Back Pain Association
Grundy House
31-33 Park Road
Teddington
Middlesex
TW11 0AB
Tel: 01 977 5474

British Limbless Ex-Servicemen's
   Association
Frankland Moore House
185/7 High Road
Chadwell Heath
Essex
RM6 6NA
Tel: 01 590 1124/5

British Migraine Association
178a High Road
Byfleet
Weybridge
Surrey
KT14 7ED
Tel: 093 23 52468

Centre on Environment for the
   Handicapped
126 Albert Street
London
NW1 7NF
Tel: 01 267 6111, Ext. 264/5

Chest, Heart and Stroke
   Association
Tavistock House North
Tavistock Square
London
WC1H 9JE
Tel: 01 387 3012

Consumers' Association
14 Buckingham Street
London
WC2N 6DS
Tel: 01 839 1222

Disability Alliance
1 Cambridge Terrace
London
NW1 4JL
Tel: 01 935 4992

Disabled Income Group
Attlee House
28 Commercial Road
London
E1 6LR
Tel: 01 247 2128/6877

Disabled Living Foundation
380/384 Harrow Road
London
W9 2HU
Tel: 01 289 6111

Greater London Association for the
    Disabled (GLAD)
1 Thorpe Close
London
W10 5XL
Tel: 01 960 5799

Greater London Association for
    Initiatives in Disablement
    (GLAID)
Flat 4
188 Ramsden Road
Balham
London
SW12
Tel: 01 673 4310

Joint Committee on Mobility for
    the Disabled
c/o ASBAH
Tavistock House North
Tavistock Square
London
WC1H 9JE
Tel: 01 388 1382

Mobility Information Service
Copthorne Community Hall
Shelton Road
Copthorne
Shrewsbury
SY3 8TD
Tel: 0743 68383

Multiple Sclerosis Society of Great
    Britain and Northern Ireland
25 Effie Road
Fulham
London
SW6 1EE
Tel: 01 381 4022/5

Patients' Association
Room 33
18 Charing Cross Road
London
WC2H 0HR
Tel: 01 240 0671

PHAB (Physically Handicapped
    and Able Bodied)
42 Devonshire Street
London
W1N 1LN
Tel: 01 637 7475

Spinal Injuries Association
Yeoman House
76 St James Lane
Muswell Hill
London
N10
Tel: 01 444 2121

Hobbies and activities

Organizations exist to give you advice, local contacts, etc.

British Ski Club for the Disabled
Corton House
Corton
Warminster
Wilts
BA12 0SZ
Tel: 0985 5321

British Sports Association for the
    Disabled
Hayward House
Ludwic Guttman Sports Centre for
    the Disabled
Harvey Road
Aylesbury
Bucks
HP21 8PP
Tel: 0296 27889

Committee for the Promotion of
    Angling for the Disabled
18–19 Claremont Crescent
Edinburgh
EH7 4QD
Tel: 031 556 3882

Committee on Sexual and Personal
    Relationships of the Disabled
Brook House
2/16 Torrington Place
London
WC1E 7HN
Tel: 01 637 4712

Cultural Society of the Disabled
10 Warwick Row
London
SW1E 5EP
Tel: 01 828 3488, Ext. 223

Disabled Drivers' Association
Ashwellthorpe Hall
Ashwellthorpe
Norwich
NR16 1EX
Tel: 050 841 449

Disabled Drivers' Insurance Bureau
(Chartwell Insurance Brokers)
292 Hale Lane
Edgware
Middlesex
HA8 8NP
Tel: 01 958 3135

Disabled Drivers' Motor Club Ltd
9 Park Parade
Gunnersbury Avenue
London
W3 9BD
Tel: 01 993 6454

Disabled Motorists' Federation
15 Rookery Road
Tilston
Malpas
Cheshire
SW14 7HE
Tel: 082 98 373

Hand Crafts Advisory Association
    for the Disabled
Room 313
31 Clerkenwell Close
London
EC1R 0AT
Tel: 01 250 1850

Handihols
12 Ormonde Avenue
Rochford
Essex
SS4 1QW
Tel: 0702 548257

Holidays for the Disabled
12 Ryle Road
Farnham
Surrey
GU9 8RW

Home Opportunities for
    Professional Employment
96 Greencroft Gardens
London NW6 3PH

National Council for Voluntary
  Organizations
26 Bedford Square
London
WC1B 3HU
Tel: 01 636 4066

Young Disabled on Holiday
6 Hampden Road
Knowle
Bristol
Tel: 0272 711655

Sources of information for specialist pain services

Pain Relief Foundation
Walton Hospital
Rice Lane
Liverpool
L9 1AE
Tel: 051 525 3611

Intractable Pain Society
Tim Nash
Honorary Secretary
IPS
Department of Anaesthetics
Basingstoke District Hospital
Basingstoke
Herts
RG24 9NA

Therapist organizations

The following organizations can give information on particular therapies, and how to obtain treatment.

British Acupuncture Association
34 Alderney Street
Westminster
London
SW1V 4EU
Tel: 01 834 1012/3353

British Chiropractice Association
5 First Avenue
Chelmsford
Essex
CM1 1RX
Tel: 0245 358487

British Homeopathic Association
27a Devonshire Street
London
W1N 1RJ
Tel: 01 935 2163

British Osteopathic Association
8-10 Boston Place
London
NW1 6QH
Tel: 01 262 5250

The British Psychological Society
St Andrews House
48 Princess Road East
Leicester
LE1 7DR
Tel: 0533 549568

British Society of Hypnotherapists
51 Queen Anne Street
London
W1M 9FA
Tel: 01 935 7075

British Society of Medical and
    Dental Hypnotists
42 Links Road
Ashtead
Surrey
Tel: 037 22 73522

Chartered Society of
    Physiotherapy
14 Bedford Row
London
WC1R 4ED
Tel: 01 242 1941

College of Occupational Therapists
20 Rede Place
off Chepstow Place
London
W2 4TV
Tel: 01 229 9738/9

College of Speech Therapists
6 Lechmere Road
London
NW2 5BU
Tel: 01 459 8521

Index